```
E          Rockwell, Anne F.
ROC        My barber /


55A3407
```

MAR 27 '84 — **DATE DUE**

```
E          Rockwell, Anne F.
ROC        My barber /


55A3407
```

DATE DUE	BORROWER'S NAME	ROOM NUMBER
JAN 17 '82	Anthony	102

Anne & Harlow Rockwell

My Barber

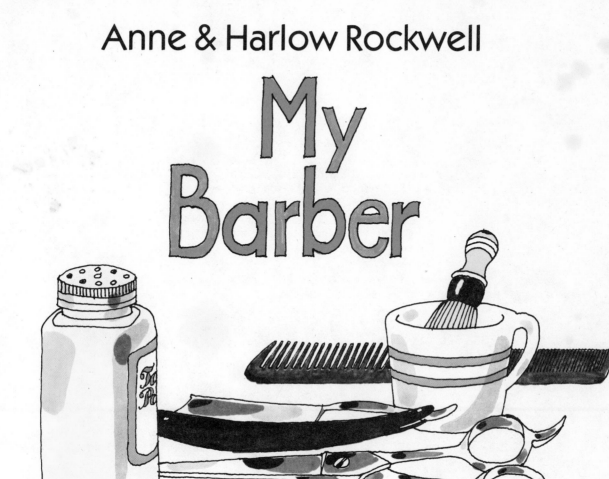

84-26

Macmillan Publishing Co., Inc., New York

Macmillan Publishing Co., Inc.
866 Third Avenue, New York, N.Y. 10022
Collier Macmillan Canada, Ltd.
Printed in the United States of America

10 9 8 7 6 5 4 3 2 1

Library of Congress Cataloging in Publication Data
Rockwell, Anne F   My barber.

  Summary: A young boy and his father visit their barbers.
  [1. Barbers—Fiction] I. Rockwell, Harlow, joint author.   II. Title.
PZ7.R5943My   [E]   80-24496   ISBN 0-02-777630-1

My mother said my hair was too long.
My father said so, too.
So I went to my barber.

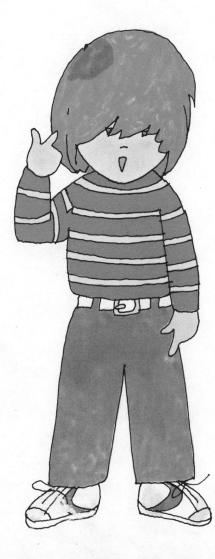

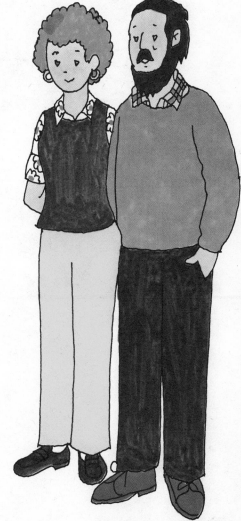

Sometimes, when I go to my barber,
I have to wait for him.
Then I look at the comic books
and watch the people
getting their hair cut.
But today my barber is not busy.
He is ready for me, so...

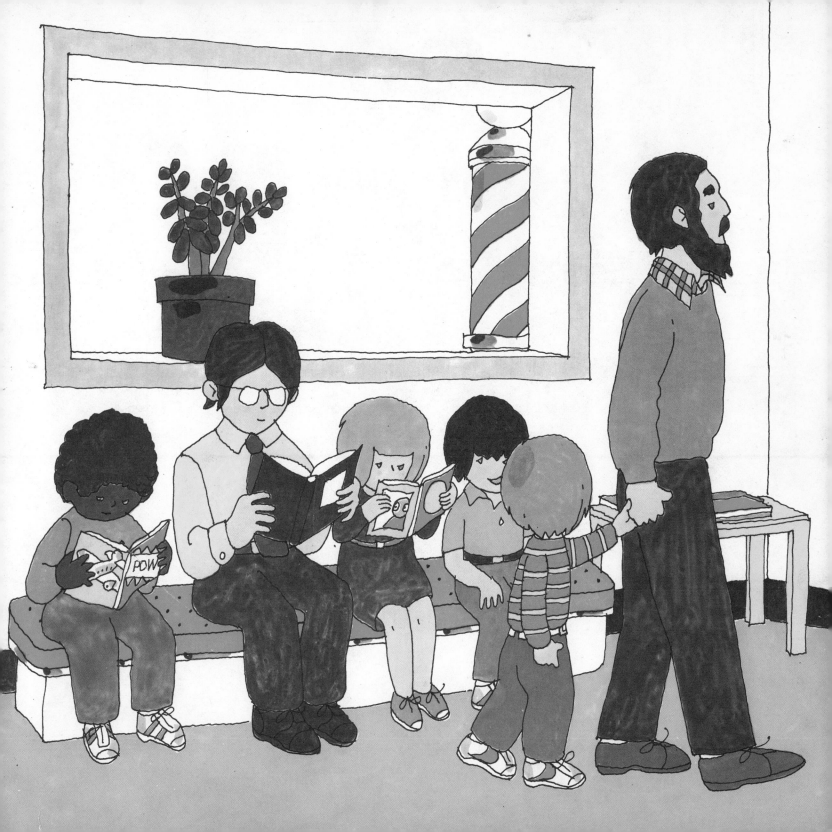

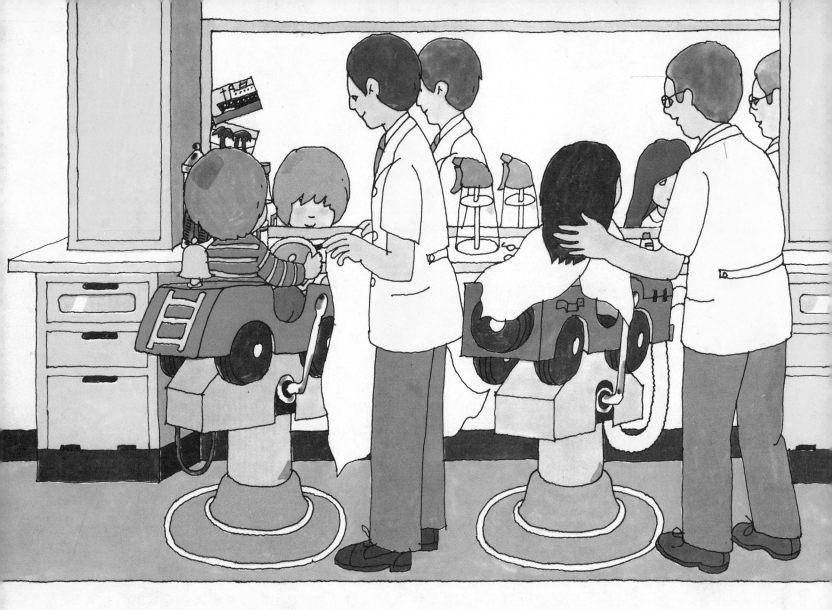

I sit in the fire engine.

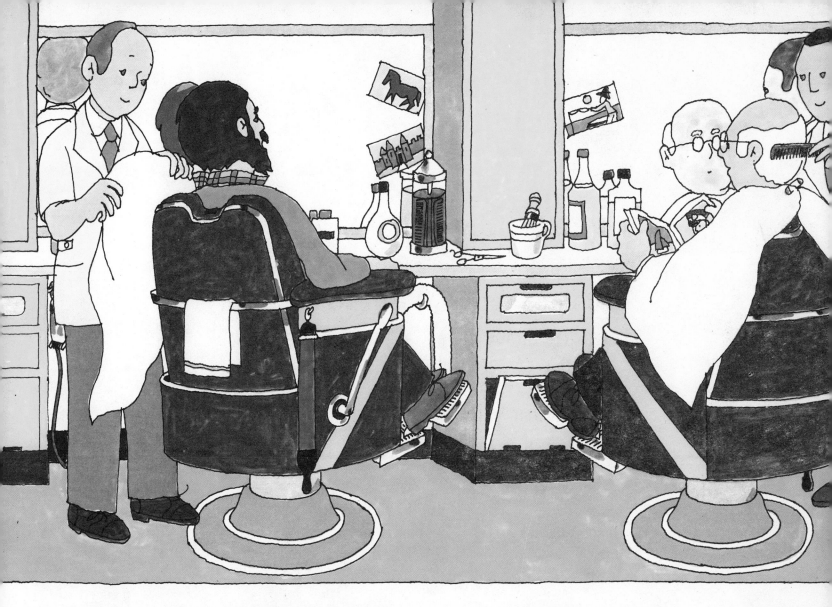

My father sits in the barber chair
that goes up and down and turns around.
He wants to have his hair cut
and his beard trimmed.

My barber covers me
with a big plastic cloth.
Then he wets my hair and combs it
straight down,
around my ears and over my eyebrows.
I look funny in the big mirror
at the barber shop.

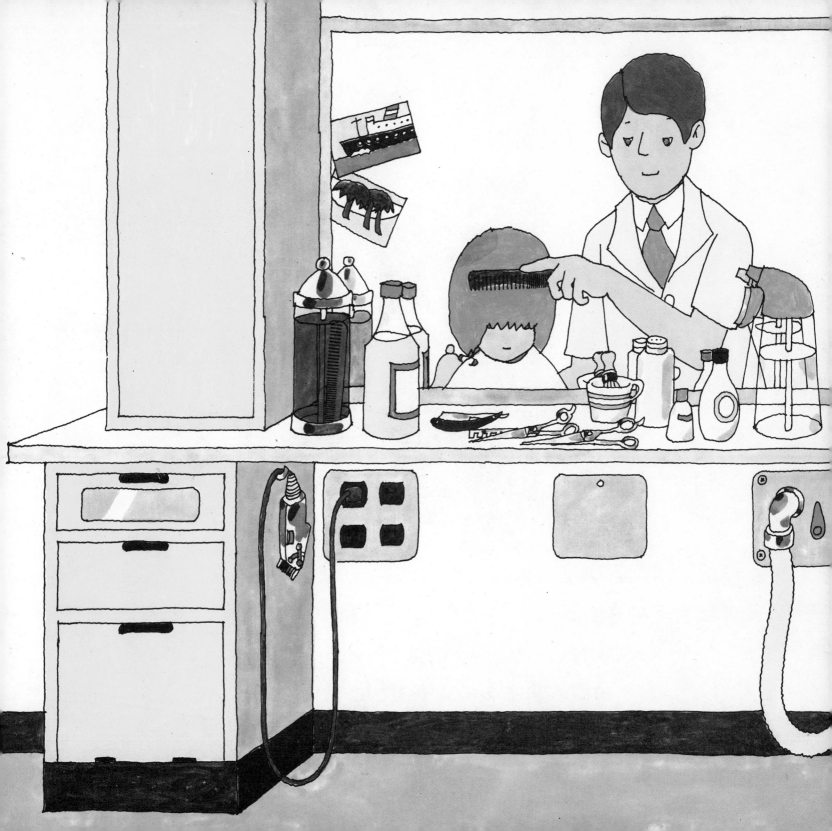

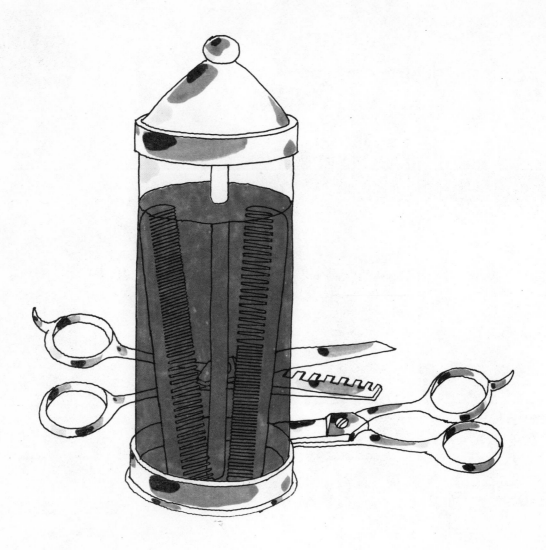

My barber keeps his combs
in a glass jar of purple liquid.
He says that makes them clean.

My barber uses sharp scissors
to cut my hair
and thinning shears
to thin it.

He has electric clippers
to trim the back of my hair.
The clippers buzz and tickle.

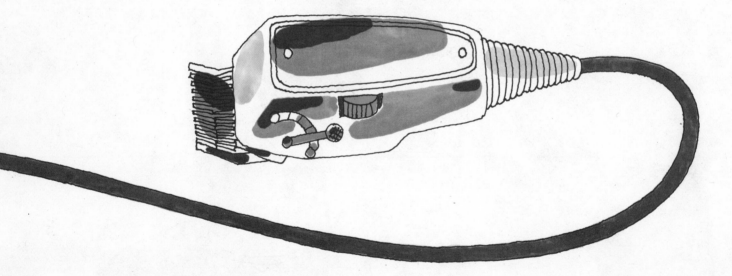

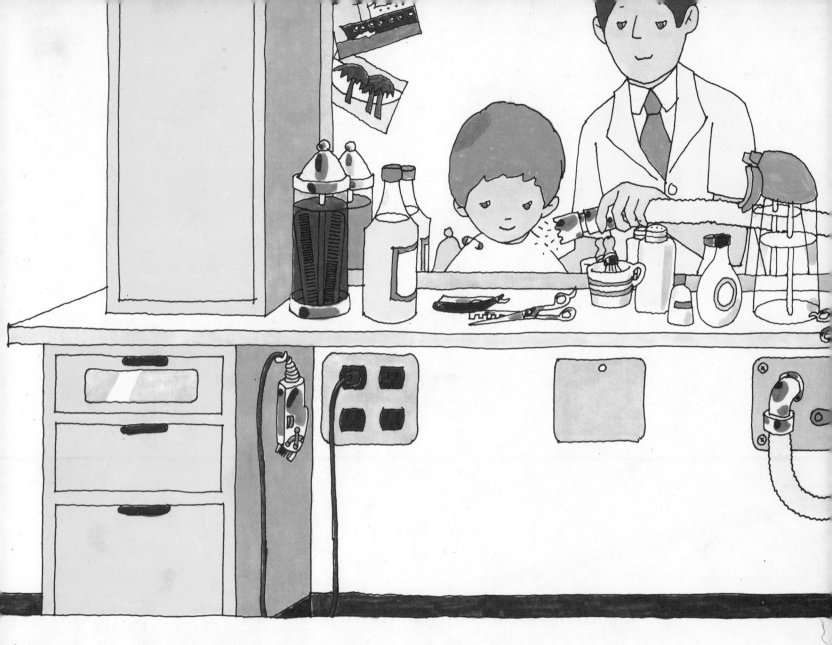

He has a vacuum cleaner tube
that comes out of the wall.
It sucks the prickly loose hair off my neck.

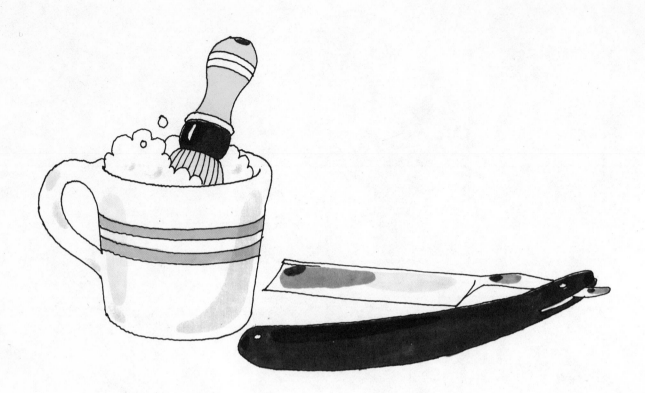

He has shaving foam and a brush
and a straight razor
to shave men's whiskers with.
But I don't have any whiskers yet!

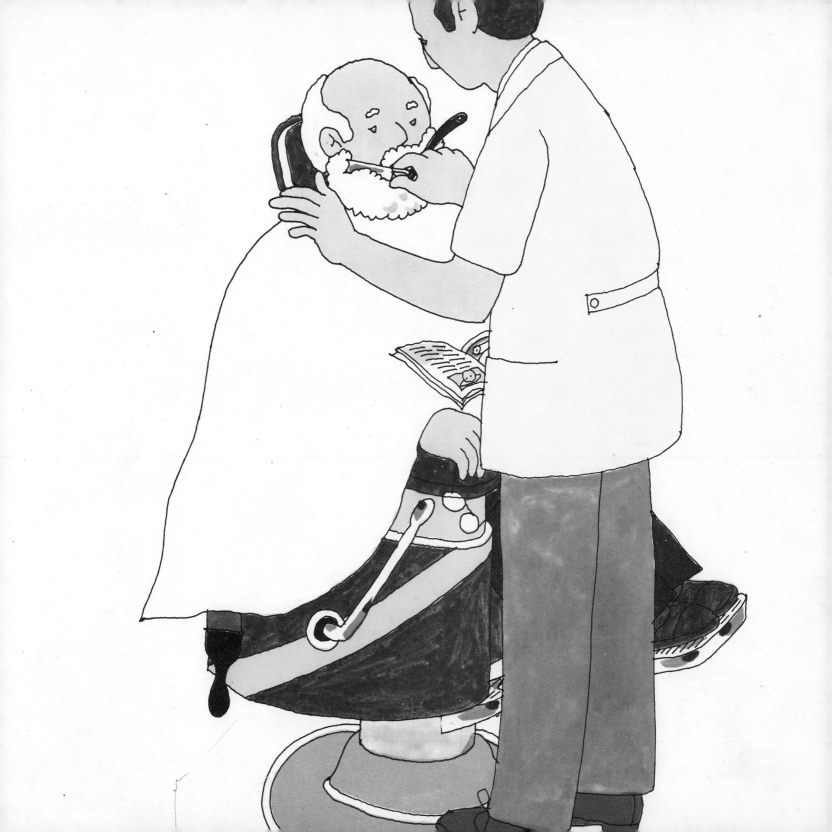

My father's barber cuts his hair
while my barber cuts mine.

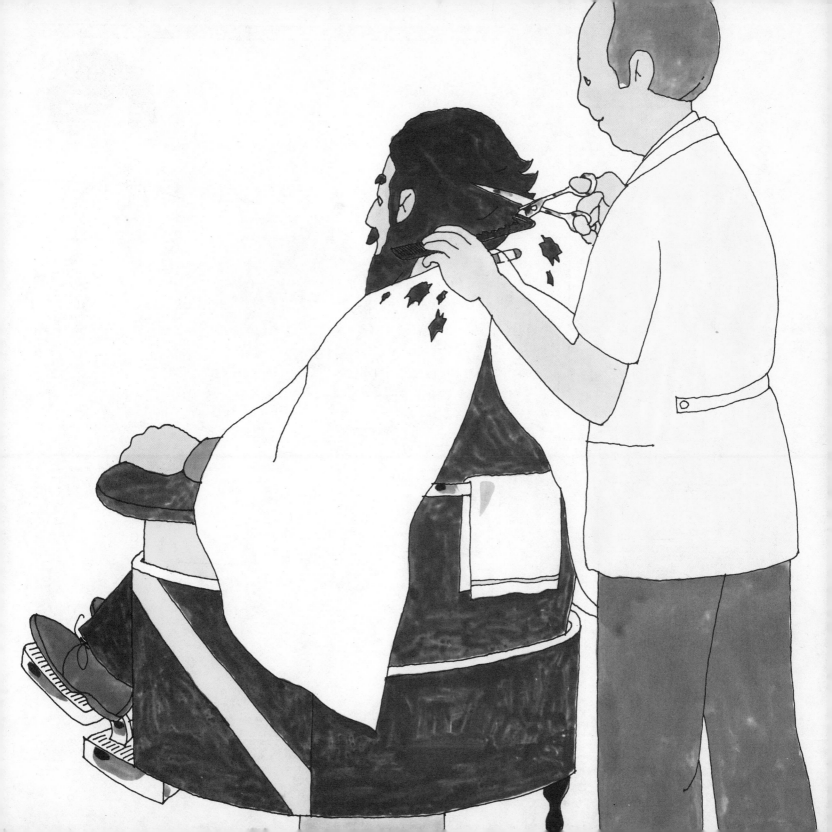

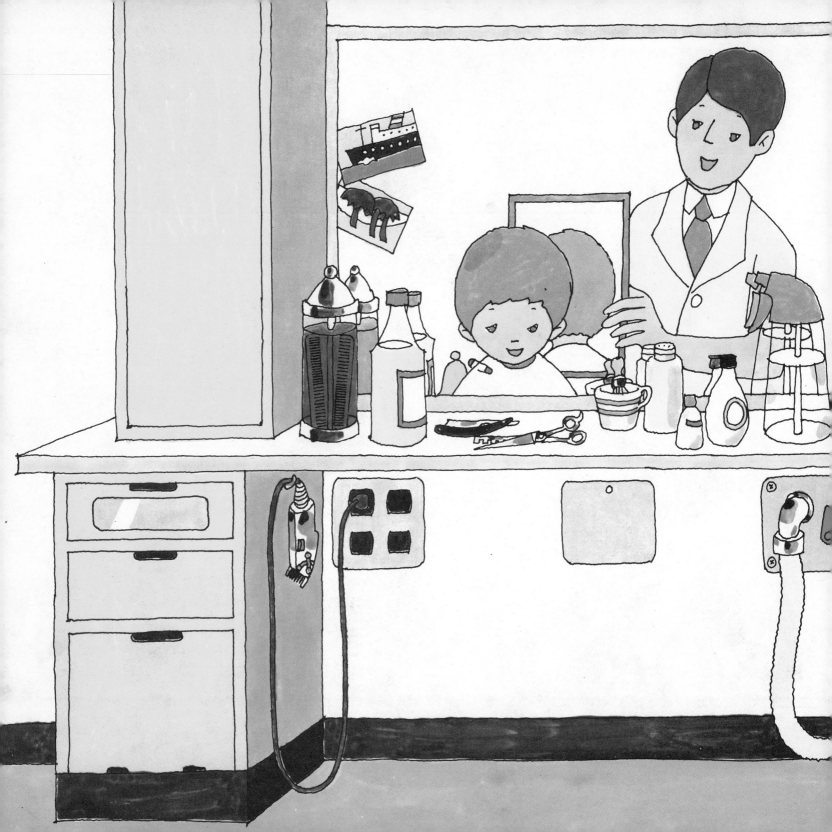

My barber holds up a mirror
so I can see
how my hair looks in back.
I like it.
It is not too short.
I tell my barber so.

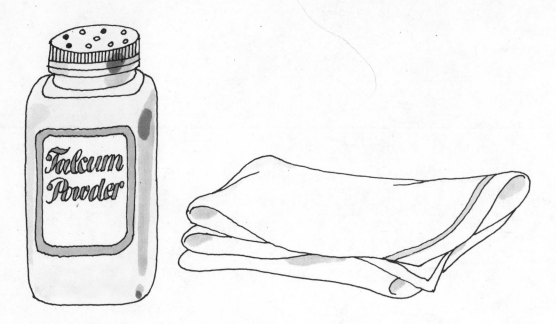

My barber has a can of talcum powder.
He sprinkles the powder on my neck
where the itchy cut hairs were.
The talcum powder smells good.

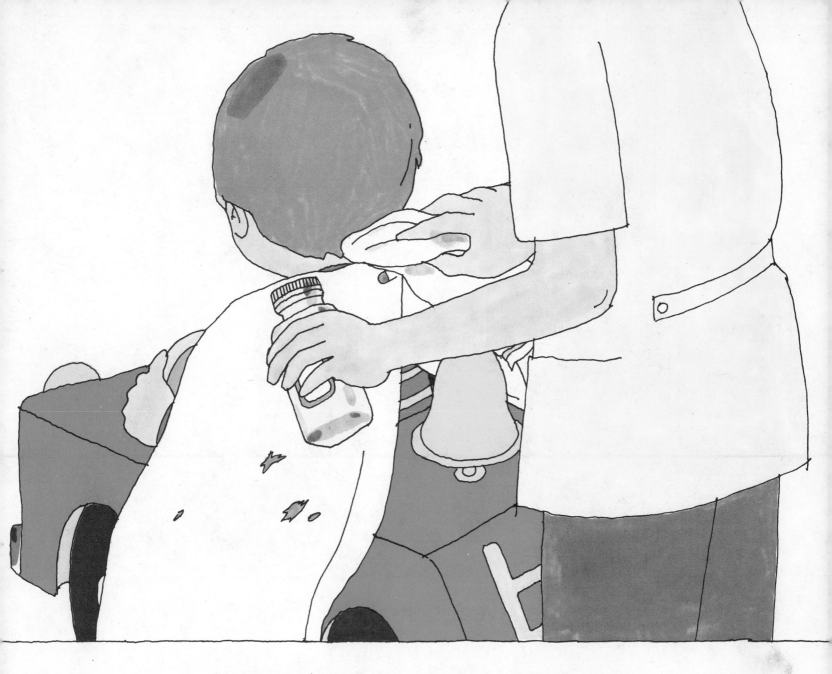

My barber uses a clean linen towel
to dust the powder off me.

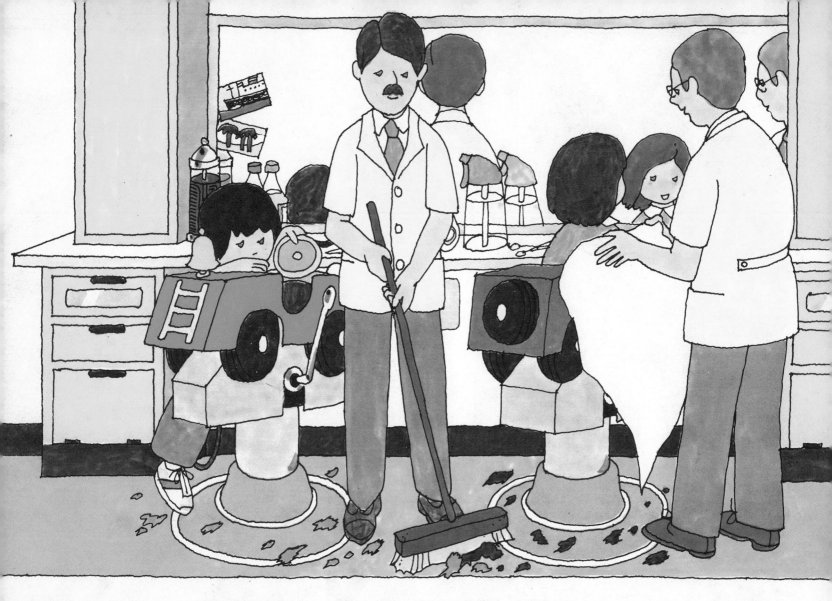

Someone sweeps the hair off the floor—
my hair, my father's hair,
the man with white hair's hair
and the hair of the girl in the jeep.

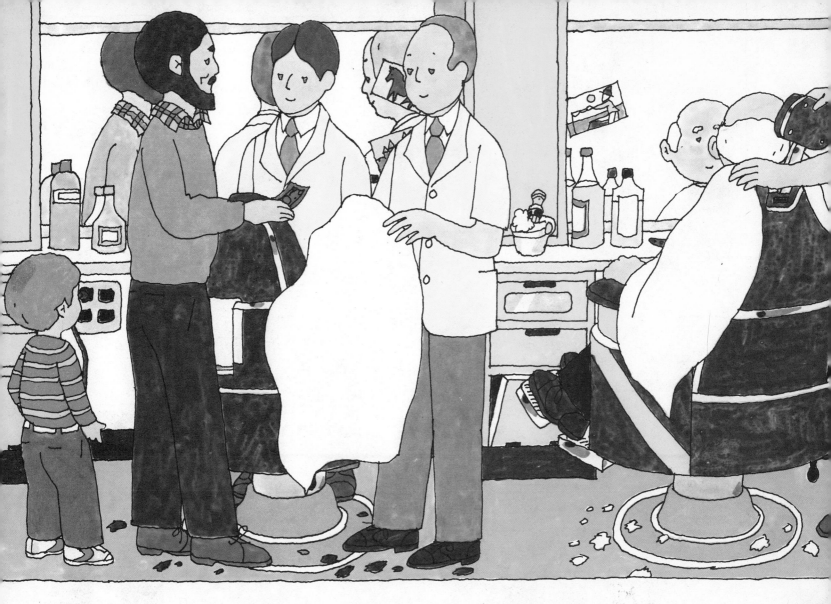

My father and I can go home now.
A boy with black hair
was waiting to sit in the fire engine.
His hair is shorter than mine was.

At home,
my mother says I look nice.
She says my father does, too.
She is right.
We do.

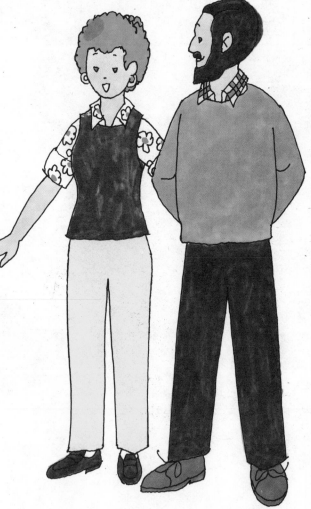
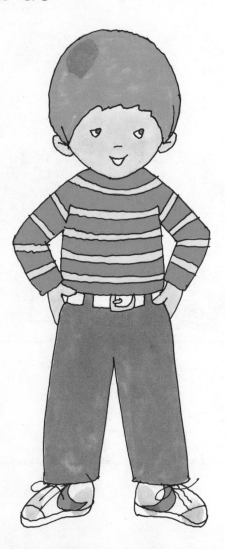